Prenatal Fitness and Health

Safe and effective options to home prenatal fitness

by

Kim Cecchi

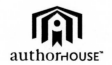

1663 LIBERTY DRIVE, SUITE 200
BLOOMINGTON, INDIANA 47403
(800) 839-8640
WWW.AUTHORHOUSE.COM

First published by AuthorHouse 07/22/05

ISBN: 1-4208-4544-6 (sc)

Library of Congress Control Number: 2005903789

Printed in the United States of America
Bloomington, Indiana

This book is printed on acid-free paper.

I would like to say a special thank-you to my model, friend of over 20 years, and sister-in-law, Jaqi Cecchi, who was pregnant with my niece Sophia when the pictures in this book were taken.

TABLE OF CONTENTS

INTRODUCTION

First of all, I would like to say congratulations! If you have picked up this book, chances are that you have recently found out that you are expecting a baby, or that you plan to start trying to conceive in the near future. Having my son, Nicholas, was the best thing that ever happened to me. He has brought so much joy to my life!

Learning how to treat your body before, during, and after you become pregnant increases your chances of having a problem-free pregnancy and birth.

In this book, I will not give lengthy explanations or go into depth with a lot of details - that is for your doctor. The purpose of this book is to give you options in your exercise routines that are safe and beneficial to both you and your baby. I will also cover the basics of prenatal nutrition, and give you a better understanding of what you and your baby need to be healthy and strong during your pregnancy.

Get permission from your doctor before beginning any of the exercises. Let him or her know which exercises you feel would work out best for you, and the two of you can work together to ensure a healthy baby and mother.

Best of Luck!
Kim Cecchi

CHAPTER ONE

Do's and don'ts of prenatal nutrition and health

PRENATAL NUTRITIONAL AND HEALTH DO'S AND DON'TS

If you have any questions about the following prenatal guidelines, please ask your doctor.

<u>DO</u>

1. Do start taking prenatal vitamins when you start trying to conceive, or as soon as you discover that you are pregnant.

   WHY? Prenatal vitamins help insure the health and growth of your baby. If you get constipated from them, try some without Iron in them - I found some at GNC. If they make you nauseous, try taking them before you go to bed.

2. Do eat foods high in fiber.

   WHY? They help reduce the risk of developing constipation and hemorrhoids.

3. Do get plenty of protein, carbohydrates and vitamin B6.

   WHY? They help reduce morning sickness and build the baby's placenta, tissues, and red blood cells in the mother.

4. Do have your meals and snacks consist of fresh fruits and vegetables, legumes, grains, and foods rich in protein and calcium.

   WHY? They are the most beneficial to you and your baby.

5. Do drink 5-6 8 ounce glasses of water or juice a day - more if you exercise.

   WHY? To keep your body well hydrated and reduce the risk of premature labor.

6. Do consume 1,000 mg. of calcium every day.

   WHY? To keep your bones and teeth strong and healthy.

7. Do consume 5-6 portions of vegetables every day. One portion is 1 cup raw, 1 half cup cooked or 1 whole piece(1 carrot).

   WHY? Vegetables supply the body with folic acid, vitamin C, phytochemicals and beta carotene, which are essential for your baby.

8. Do consume 3-4 portions of fruit. One portion is 1 cup of whole berries or 1 piece (apple).

   WHY? They are packed with vitamins and minerals essential to a healthy pregnancy.

9. Do consume 6-7 portions of grains. One portion is 1 slice of bread, ½ bagel, or ½ cup of cooked pasta, rice or cereal.

   WHY? They contain chromium, iron, selenium some of the B vitamins, and fiber.

10. Do eat extra-lean meats and skinless poultry (3 oz. Portions).

    WHY? To help control your fat consumption.

11. Do eat small meals or snacks every three to four hours.

    WHY? To keep your energy level elevated and to prevent overeating at mealtimes.

12. Do have your caloric intake between 2,000 and 2,500 a day during your first trimester.

    WHY? During the first trimester your caloric needs remain about the same as before.

13. Do eat 300 extra calories a day(more if exercising) during the second and third trimesters.

   WHY? As the baby grows your body needs more calories to keep up with the growth.

14. Do limit extra fat calories to 25 to 30 percent of your total daily calories.

   WHY? Your body will store the extra fat in places that you do not want it.

15. Do read labels on food to determine their fat and calorie content.

   WHY? You will be able to make better food choices if you know what is in it.

16. Do have regular dental check-ups.

   WHY? Keeping your teeth and gums healthy will help prevent gum disease.

17. Do brush your teeth twice daily and floss once a day.

   WHY? Brushing and flossing will help prevent gum disease.

18. Do call your doctor if you have any bleeding or cramping.

   WHY? These could be a sign of a problem and should be addressed immediately.

19. Do avoid emotional stress.

   WHY? Stress can raise blood pressure and repress appetite, both of which are bad for the baby.

20. Do keep your weight gain between 25 and 35 pounds if you are average in weight.

WHY? Too much or too little weight gain can cause problems for you and the baby.

21. Do eat and drink more if your exercise.

WHY? Exercise depletes your energy and dehydrates you.

22. Do moisturize your skin daily - especially your belly.

WHY? Dry skin is itchy and uncomfortable.

23. Do wear a supportive bra.

WHY? To prevent ligament damage, sagging and pain in your breasts.

24. Do bend at the knees when lifting something off the floor.

WHY? Bending at the waist could injure your back.

25. Do sit with your back straight - use a stability ball when you can.

WHY? Good posture helps prevent back problems.

26. Do lay on your left side when sleeping or resting.

WHY? This is the best position to insure maximum blood flow to you and the baby.

Lying on your back causes the uterus to press on the inferior vena cava which carries oxygenated blood to the heart. You may develop supine hypotensive syndrome, which involves nausea, dizziness, claustrophobia and breathing difficulties, if you lie on your back after your first trimester.

27. Do get Thimerosol-free Rhogam injections if you have a negative blood type.

WHY? Thimerosol is a preservative that is almost 50 percent ethyl mercury.

DON'T

1. Don't smoke.

WHY? It is unhealthy for you and the baby. Women who smoke during their pregnancy often have lower birth-weight babies.

2. Don't drink alcohol.

WHY? Drinking alcohol can cause fetal alcohol syndrome and damage to the baby.

3. Don't take any drugs unless they are prescribed by your doctor.

WHY? Non-prescription drugs may harm your baby or you.

4. Don't think of your pregnancy as a time to eat whatever you want - now is the perfect time to start eating better!

WHY? Excess weight gain can lead to health problems, such as diabetes, and it makes losing the weight post-partum more difficult.

5. Don't skip breakfast.

WHY? You will have less energy, and possible morning sickness and headaches.

6. Don't drink caffeinated beverages.

WHY? They are diuretics and consumption can lead to dehydration.

7. Don't eat candy or candied fruit.

    WHY? They supply few nutrients and are high in sugar.

8. Don't eat cereal sweetened with sugar.

    WHY? They are high in sugar and fat, and supply few nutrients.

9. Don't eat cookies, brownies, pies, etc.

    WHY? They have a lot of sugar and calories and are low on nutritional value.

10. Don't eat snack foods like potato chips that are high in salt.

    WHY? Salt makes you retain water.

11. Don't eat tuna, shark, mackerel, tilefish, swordfish, bluefish, striped bass, sea bass, halibut marlin or pike.

    WHY? They have a high mercury content.

12. Don't sit in hot tubs or saunas.

    WHY? The high temperatures cause your body temperature to rise, and can impede the development of your baby. Raising your body temperature for long periods can cause birth defects and even death.

13. Don't have x-rays done.

    WHY? X-rays contain ionizing radiation, which can harm your baby in large doses.

14. Don't drink herbal tea unless your doctor says it is safe.

    WHY? Some herbs can cause an allergic reaction, some are toxic, and others are potent enough to be considered drugs.

15. Don't lie on your back after the first trimester.

WHY? The weight of the uterus presses on the vena cava, cutting off the oxygenated blood supply to you and the baby.

16. Don't wear high heels.

WHY? To avoid accidents as your body becomes larger. Your center of gravity shifts and your balance is not always great.

17. Don't sit or stand for long periods of time.

WHY? To avoid leg swelling and back pain.

18. Don't cross your legs when sitting in a chair.

WHY? This cuts off circulation to the legs and can strain your back.

19. Don't have mercury fillings added or removed.

WHY? It could get into your blood and harm the baby.

CHAPTER TWO

Do's and Don'ts of Prenatal Exercise

PRENATAL EXERCISE DO'S AND DON'TS

<u>DO</u>

1. Do take a daily prenatal vitamin and eat healthy.

   WHY? To ensure that you and your baby have the nutrients you need.

2. Do get your doctors approval before you begin any exercise program.

   WHY? For safety. They know your body and limitations the best.

3. Do keep cool and hydrated.

   WHY? Overheating can lead to fainting, and dehydration can lead to pre-mature labor.

4. Do rise slowly.

   WHY? To prevent dizziness and loss of balance.

5. Do stop exercising when you feel fatigued.

   WHY? To prevent fainting and exhaustion.

6. Do check for Diastasis Recti after 20 weeks(Chapter 3).

   WHY? To determine if you have a separation in your abdominal wall.

7. Do eat before exercising.

   WHY? To keep your energy level up.

8. Do wear footwear with ankle and arch support.

   WHY? To prevent injuries and falls.

9. Do relax often.

   WHY? Relaxation during pregnancy can decrease your risk of having a hyperactive child and can aid you in labor by reducing the need for pain medication.

10. Do your Kegels every day - several times.

    WHY? To keep your pelvic floor strong for childbirth.

11. Do walk whenever you can.

    WHY? It keeps your weight gain minimized, keeps the legs strong, and increases circulation.

12. Do practice good posture - especially when you exercise.

    WHY? To prevent falling over and injuring yourself.

13. Do wear a supportive bra.

    WHY? To prevent ligament damage and sagging.

14. Do wear comfortable, non-binding clothing.

    WHY? No explanation needed!

DON'T

1. Don't exercise in a prone position(on your belly).

    WHY? Because you might injure the baby or the uterus.

2. Don't exercise in a supine position(on your back).

    WHY? Blood flow in the vena cava will be cut off.

3. Don't do twisting exercises.

    WHY? You can cause damage to the uterus and surrounding ligaments or your back.

4. Don't do jumping exercises.

    WHY? You can cause damage to the uterus and increase your chances of falling.

5. Don't do inversions(upside down).

    WHY? The placenta at the top of the uterus can dislodge and the umbilical cord can twist.

6. Don't do backbends or back extensions.

    WHY? To prevent injuries to the uterus by having too much lumbar spine pressure.

7. Don't do balances without support.

    WHY? You will increase your chances of a fall if unsupported.

8. Don't hold your breath.

    WHY? This will prevent the baby from getting oxygen and possibly lead to you fainting.

9. Don't do full lunges after the first trimester.

   WHY? They are not stable and are bad for the knees.

10. Don't elevate the heart-rate above 140 or longer than 30 minutes without your doctor's approval.

    WHY? Increased oxygen requirements and breathing problems during pregnancy leave less oxygen available for aerobic exercise.

11. Don't overstretch - only stretch to the point of mild tension.

    WHY? Over-stretching leads to muscle pulls.

12. Don't do exercises that strain your joints.

    WHY? It leads to injuries.

13. Don't make rapid changes in direction.

    WHY? Your balance is compromised and falls need to be avoided.

14. Don't do ballistic(fast) movements.

    WHY? Again, your balance is compromised.

15. Don't use resistance when working abductors and adductors(inner and outer thighs).

    WHY? The hormone Relaxin makes the ligaments soft and prone to injury.

16. Don't mis-align the wrists.

    WHY? To prevent injury, especially if you develop Carpal Tunnel Syndrome.

17. Don't do deep flexions or extensions.

    WHY? To prevent injury to soft joints.

18. Don't continue exercising if you are having a Braxton Hicks contraction. Stop, then resume exercising after the contraction passes.

    WHY? The contraction will distract you from doing the exercise correctly and could lead to injury.

19. Don't exercise to lose weight.

    WHY? Losing weight while pregnant prevents the baby from getting the nutrients it needs to grow.

20. Don't try to exceed pre-pregnancy fitness levels.

    WHY? Exceeding fitness levels now can cause damage or injury to you or the baby.

21. Don't exercise on rocky terrain or unstable ground.

    WHY? The possibility of falling is too risky.

22. Don't do activities that put increased risk to mother and baby - contact sports, skiing, etc.

    WHY? Injuries and loss of the baby are too great.

23. Don't push your body to the maximum.

    WHY? Injuries can occur to you or the baby.

CHAPTER THREE

Diastasis Recti

DIASTASIS RECTI

Diastasis Recti is a condition caused by your expanding uterus where the muscles in your abdominal wall separate. This condition is not dangerous to you or your baby, but should be prevented if possible. Doing the abdominal exercises located in the balance ball chapter of this book will help prevent it from developing and also help if you already have it. You should start checking for this condition regularly after you are 20 weeks along in your pregnancy. Diastasis often heals itself after childbirth.

To see if you have developed Diastasis Recti, perform the following test on yourself:

Lie down on your back with your shoulders raised up on a pillow and your knees bent. Place the fingertips of your index and middle fingers about an inch below your navel. Lift your head and feel if you have soft tissue or a ridge in your abdominal wall. If you do, that is diastasis.

If you do not have a balance ball to use, you can try a modified abdominal crunch - If you are past 12 weeks, prop your torso up with pillows to raise your shoulders above your belly.

Wrap a towel around your waist and gently cross it in front without knotting it. Grasp and pull the ends up and out slightly as you contract your abdominal muscles and raise your head as you exhale. Leave your shoulders down.

CHAPTER FOUR

Warm-up

WARM-UP

STANDING - Feet shoulder width apart, knees soft, belly in, arms at your sides

1. Neck - Lift the chin up toward the ceiling, back to neutral, down to your chest, and back to neutral. Repeat 3 more times. Then tilt the left ear toward the left shoulder, back to neutral, tilt the right ear toward the right shoulder, and back to neutral. Repeat 3 more times.

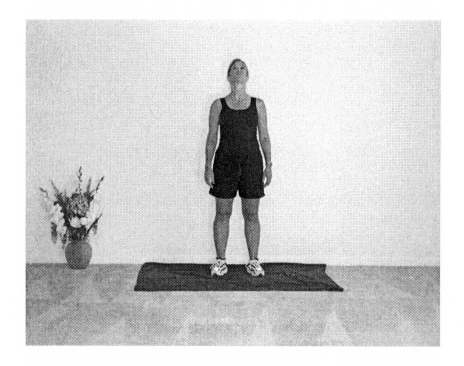

2. Shoulders - Raise both shoulders up toward the ears, then back down. Repeat 3 more times. Lift the shoulders up and roll them back and around. Repeat 3 more times. Then reverse the circle and bring the shoulders up and roll them forward and around. Repeat 3 more times.

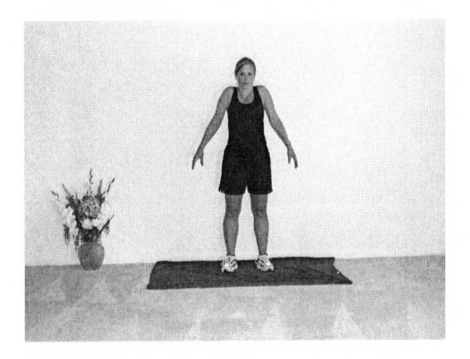

3. Back - Place your hands on your knees. Inhale, raise the head and chest. Exhale, pull the belly in, round the back and drop the head. Repeat 3 more times.

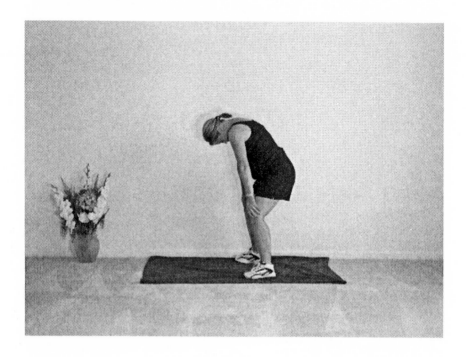

MOVING (no pictures)

4. March in place for 16 counts.

5. Bring your knees out(opening the hips) and to the side and march for 16 counts.

6. March in place for 16 counts.

7. Walk forward and back - Step right, left, right, left heel forward. Walk backward left, right, left, right heel forward. After four repetitions add chest presses by bringing the hands to chest level, pressing them forward until arms are straight, then bring them back to the chest. Do one chest press for every two steps. Repeat 4 times.

8. March in place for 16 counts.

9. Grapevine - Step right, step behind the right foot with the left, and step right, bring left heel to the side. Step left, step behind the left foot with the right, step left, and bring the right heel to the side. Repeat 3 more times. Next, add lateral raises by raising the arms to the side until they reach shoulder level. Do one raise for every two steps. Do 4 times.

10. March in place for 16 counts.

11. Step-together - Step to the right, bring the left foot over to meet it, step left, then bring the right foot over to meet it. Do 8 counts. With a straight back and abdominals pulled in,

bend your knees and lower yourself down a few inches, keeping constant tension on the quadriceps(thighs). Repeat 16 times.

12. Stand back up and step side to side for 16 counts.

13. Hamstring Curl - Still stepping side-to-side, pull the left heel up to your buttocks, squeezing the left hamstring as you do, put left foot down, then curl the right heel up to the buttocks, and lower down. Do both legs 8 times. Now work the upper back by bringing the arms in front of you at chest level, then pull the elbows back, squeezing the shoulder blades together, and returning them to the front. Do both legs 8 times.

14. March in place for 16 counts.

15. Heel Tap Front - Extend right leg forward and bring the right heel to the floor, bring it back to meet the left leg, extend the left leg forward and bring the heel to the floor, and then bring it back to meet the right. Do 8 counts on each leg. Now add front raises by bringing the hands in front of the thighs, then as you bring the heel forward, raise, your arms in front of you until they are shoulder level, and bring them down as the heel comes back. Do 8 counts on each leg.

16. Heel Tap Side - From Heel Tap Front, bring the heels and arms out to the side, doing the same motion as to the front. Do 8 or 16 counts on each leg.

17. March in place for 16 counts.

CHAPTER FIVE

Step

1. Basic Step - Face the step and stand in the center. Stand tall and hold the belly in. Step the right foot onto the step, then the left. Feet should be shoulder width apart. Now, step down to the floor with the right foot, then the left(think...right, left, right, left). Arms can either hang at your sides or move them back and forth as if you are jogging. Do 4 slow, then 2 or 3 faster sets of 8. Repeat on left leg.

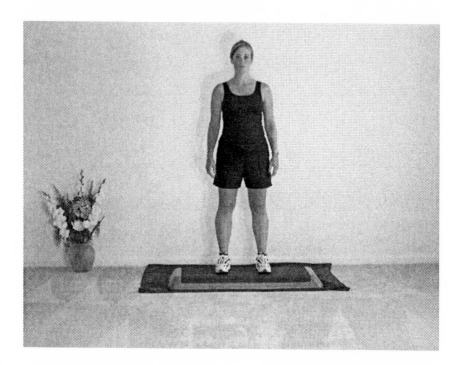

2. V-Step - Face the step and stand in the center. Stand tall and hold the belly in. Step up with the right foot and place it on top of the right side of the step, then step your left foot onto the top left side of the step. Extend the arm out to the side as the same leg steps up, and bring it down as you step back onto the floor. Step down to the floor in the center with the right foot, then the left (think ... right, left, right, left). Do 4 slow, breathing deeply during the slow reps, then do 2 or 3 faster sets of 8. Repeat on left leg.

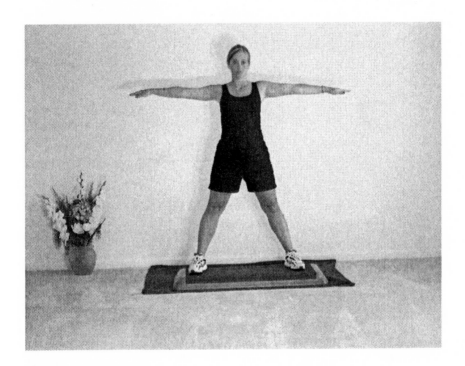

3. Up-Tap - Face the step and stand in the center. Stand tall and hold the belly in. Step up with the right foot and place it on top of the right side of the step, then bring your left foot up to tap the step right next to the right foot. Now, step far left on the step, then tap the right foot next to the left. Next, step down to the floor on the right end of the step, tap, then step far left, and tap. Swing your arms to the right as you step right, and swing them left as you move left. Do 4 slow, breathing deeply during the slow reps, then do 2 or 3 faster sets of 8. Repeat on left leg.

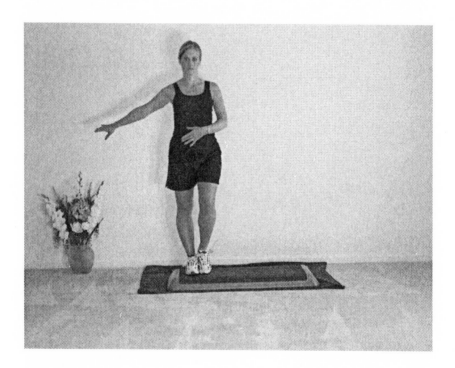

4. Leg Curl - Face the step and stand in the center. Step up with your right foot, then curl the left heel up to your left buttock, keeping the knees in line and squeezing the hamstring as you pull it. Step down to the floor in the center with your left foot, then step down with the right foot (think...step, curl, down, down). As you curl the leg, do a biceps curl to the front by bending the elbows and bringing the hands up to the shoulders, and lowering them as you step down. Do 4 slow, breathing deeply during the slow reps, then do 2 or 3 faster sets of 8. Repeat on left leg.

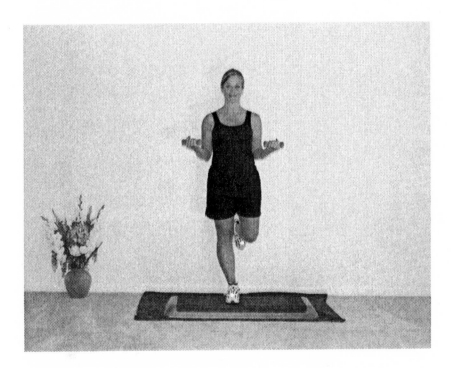

5. Back Hip Extension - Face the step and stand in the center. Step up with the right leg, extend and lift the left leg behind you and up a few inches off the floor. Step down to the floor in the center with the left foot, then step down with the right foot (think...step, lift, down, down). The arms should do a front raise as you lift the back leg by raising the arms to the front until they reach shoulder level, then lower them as you step down. Do 4 slow, breathing deeply during the slow reps, then do 2 or 3 faster sets of 8. Repeat on left leg.

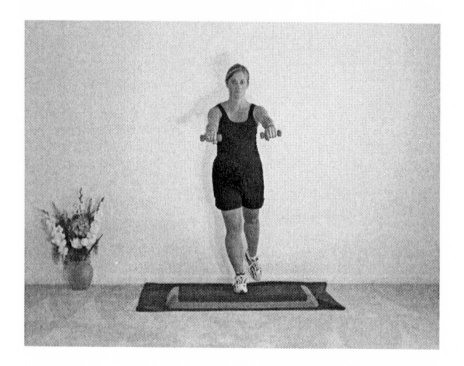

6. Side Leg Lift - Stand at the left side of your step. Step up onto the step with your right foot, raise your straight left leg up to the side until it is close to parallel with the floor. Step down to the floor with the left foot, then tap down with the right foot (think...step, lift, down, down). Your arms should do a lateral raise as you lift the left leg by raising the arms to the side until they reach shoulder level, then lower them as you step down. Do 4 slow, breathing deeply during the slow reps, then do 2 or 3 faster sets of 8. Repeat on right side.

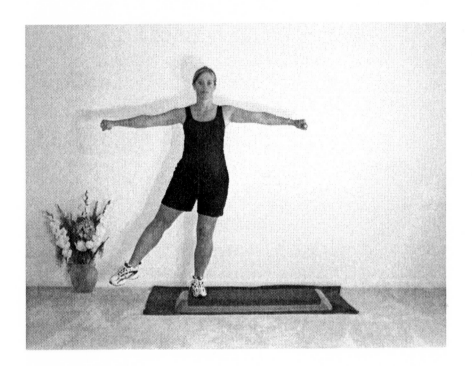

CHAPTER SIX

Exercise Band Training

These exercises can be done with a band with or without a handle.

Major muscles worked - Biceps

1. Biceps Curls - Stand in the center of the band with one handle in each hand. Your palms should be facing forward and your elbows should stay tucked in by your sides throughout the exercise. Inhale, then on the exhalation, squeeze your biceps and bring the handles up to the shoulders. Slowly lower the handles back down to the start position. You can do both arms at the same time, or one arm at a time. Do 2 or 3 sets of 8-12.

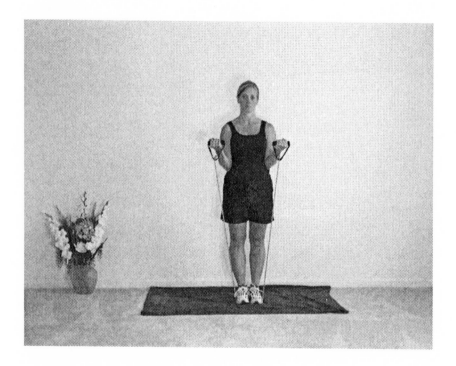

Major muscles worked - Quadriceps, Abductors and Gluteals

2. Leg Abduction/Squat Combo - Stand in the center of the band with one handle in each hand. Hold your belly in and your back straight. Step to the right, sit down and back as if sitting in a chair, press back up and bring the feet back together. Do 1 or 2 sets of 8, then do the other side.

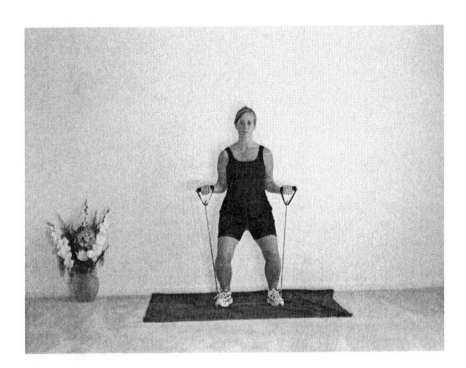

Major muscles worked - Deltoids

3. Upright Row - Stand in the center of the band. Bring both handles together by your belly and hold with both hands. Pull your belly in, keep the knees soft and your back straight. Inhale, then leading with the elbows, exhale and raise the handles up to your chin. Slowly lower back to the start position. Do 1 or 2 sets of 8. Once the belly starts getting big, take the left foot out and place it behind you to form a lunge position.

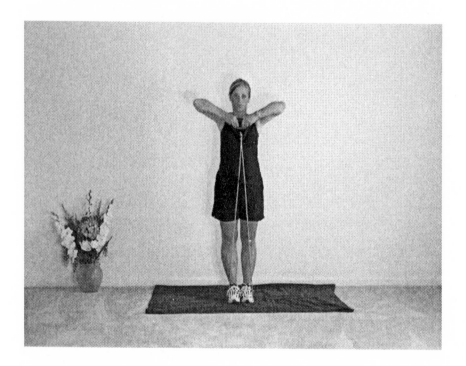

Major muscles worked - Deltoids

4. One-arm Shoulder Press - Drop the left handle to the ground, lift your right foot, then slide the band to the right until your right foot is on the band next to the handle. Your left foot should be set behind you. Bring the right hand with the handle in it up to your right shoulder. Inhale, and, keeping the elbow in line with the shoulder, exhale and press the handle up overhead. Slowly return to start position. Do 1 or 2 sets of 8, then do the other arm.

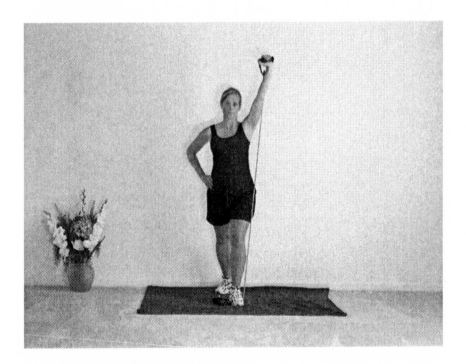

Major muscles worked - Triceps

5. Over-head Triceps Extension - Start in the same start position as #4. Bend the right elbow and bring it next to your right ear, pointing it up to the ceiling. Your right palm should also be facing the ceiling. Inhale, then exhale and extend the handle toward the ceiling until the right arm is straight. Slowly return to the start position. Keep the elbow close to the ear throughout the movement. Do 1 or 2 sets of 8, then do other arm.

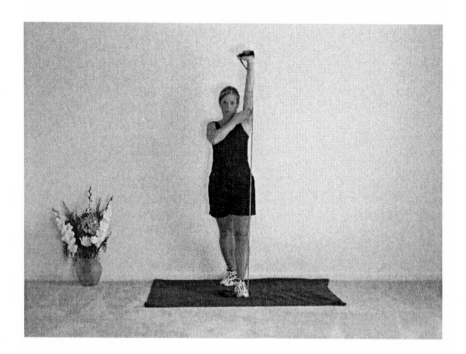

Major muscles worked - Latissimus dorsi

6. Lat Pulldown - Hold the band lengthwise in front of you and grab it, palms down, next to the handles. Wrap the band around each hand one time. Raise the band above your head. Widen your legs until they are 1 or 2 feet apart, knees soft, and belly pulled in. Inhale, then on the exhalation, pull the band down behind your head until it reaches the shoulder blades. Slowly return to start position. Do 1or 2 sets of 8.

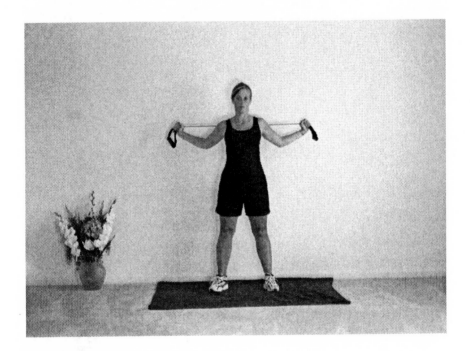

Major muscles worked - Pectorals

7. Fly - Start in same start position as #6. Pull the band down behind the head to the shoulder blades with a slight bend in the elbows. Inhale, then on the exhalation, bring the handles together in front of your chest, squeezing your pectorals as you do. Slowly return to start position. Do 1 or 2 sets of 8.

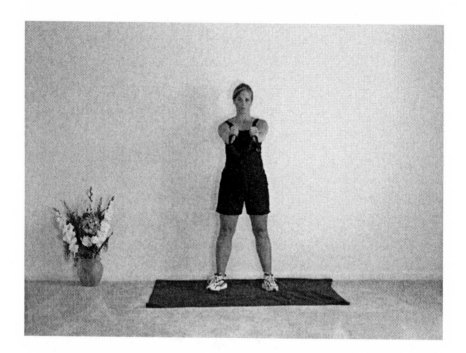

CHAPTER SEVEN

Balance Ball

Major muscles worked - Abdominals and pelvic floor

1. Abdominal Contraction and Kegels - Sit on top of the ball with your legs wide apart and feet flat on the floor, knees bent. Sit up tall, draw your naval in toward your spine, and hold. At the same time, squeeze your pelvic floor muscles by pretending that you are stopping the flow of urine. DO NOT hold your breath. Hold both contractions for 30-60 seconds. Repeat the contraction 2-3 times. Do this series several times a day if you can.

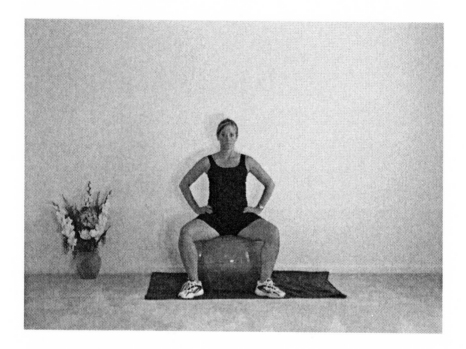

Major muscles worked - Abdominals

2. Pelvic Tilt - Sitting on top of the ball with feet wide and your hands on your hips, pull your naval into your spine. Inhale as you push your pelvis backward, then on the exhale pull the pelvis forward. Do 8-16 repetitions.

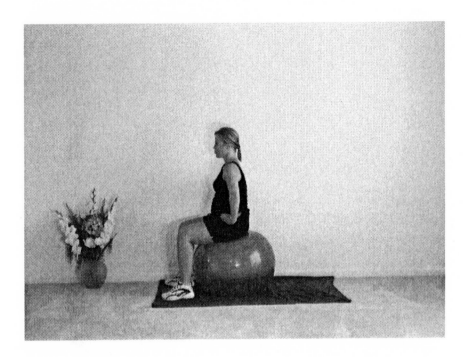

Major muscles worked - Obliques

3. Hip Lift - Sit on top of the ball with your feet wide and your hands on your hips, pull your naval into your spine. Lift your left hip off the ball, return to center, then lift the right hip off the ball, and return to center position. Do 4-8 repetitions.

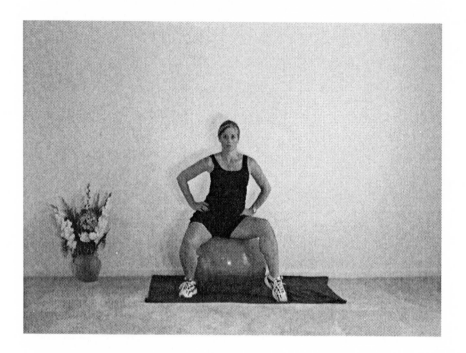

Major muscles worked - Abdominals, obliques

4. Pelvic Circles - Sit on top of the ball with the feet wide and your hands on your hips, pull your naval into your spine. Pull the pelvis forward, push the left hip to the left, circle to the back, then push your right hip to the right. Complete the circle by returning to the start position. Do 4-8 circles to the left and 4-8 circles to the right.

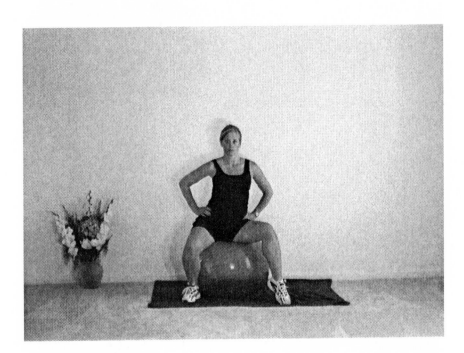

Major muscles worked - Quadriceps and hip flexors

5. Straight-leg lift - Sit on top of the ball with your feet shoulder-width apart and your hands on your hips or on the ball by your buttocks. Extend your right leg in front of you. Inhale, then on the exhalation, raise the right leg until it meets the left knee, then lower it down to the start position. Do 2 or 3 sets of 8-12, then do the left leg. You can also do these with your knee bent.

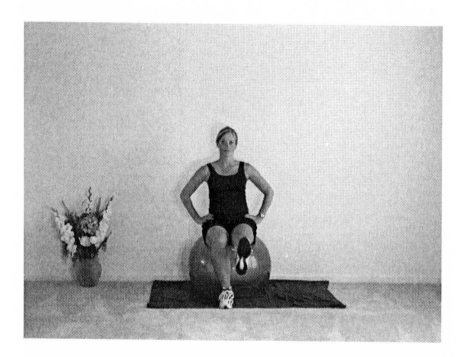

Major muscles worked - Abductors

6. Inner Thigh Lift - Sit on top of the ball with your feet shoulder-width apart and your hands on the ball by your buttocks. Let your right knee fall out to the right and bring your right foot in front of your left foot. Inhale, then on the exhalation, lift your right foot up until your right foot is even with your left knee. Lower back to the start position. Do 1 or 2 sets of 8-12, then do the left leg.

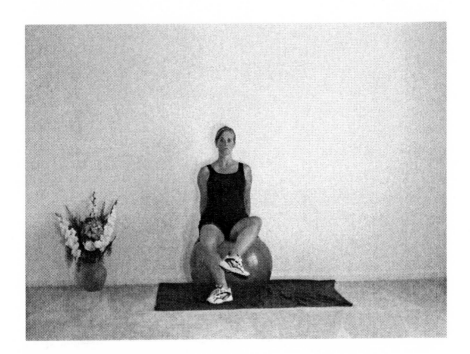

Major muscles worked - Quadriceps, Hamstrings

7. Leg Extension/Hamstring Curl - Sit on top of the ball with your feet shoulder-width apart and your hands by your chest with your palms facing out. Inhale, and lift your right knee up a few inches. Exhale and extend the foot forward to straighten the leg, and at the same time press the hands forward until the arms are straight. Retract the hands and foot back, squeezing the hamstring, and lower it down to the start position. Do 1 or 2 sets of 8-12, then do the left leg.

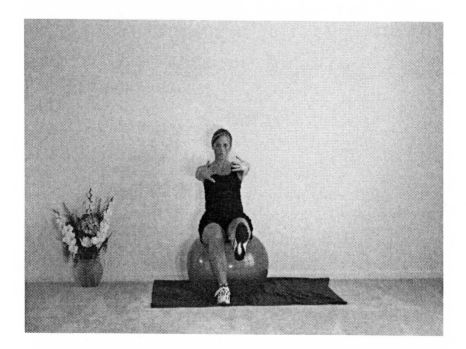

Major muscles worked - Quadriceps, Gluteals

8. Ball Squats - Stand next to a wall and place the ball against it. Turn your body to face away from the ball and lean your lower back against it. Place your hands on your hips and your feet shoulder-width apart. Make sure that your feet are out far enough so that when you squat down, your knees will not go over your toes. Inhale, and bend your knees, lowering your buttocks toward the floor until your knees are at, or close to, a 90 degree angle. Exhale, then press back up to the start position. Do 2 sets of 8-12.

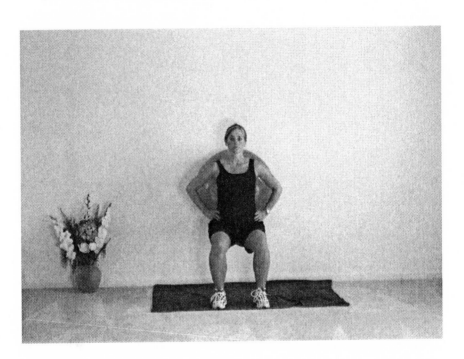

Major muscles worked - Quadriceps, Gluteals

9. Wide-leg Squats - Stand with your back against the ball at a wall. Step your feet apart about 6 to 12 inches past shoulder-width. Make sure that they are far enough apart so that when you lower down, your knees will not go over your toes. Pull your belly in and squeeze your pelvic floor muscles. Inhale, then lower your buttocks down until the knees are at, or close to, a 90 degree angle. Exhale, then press back up to the start position. Do 2 sets of 8-12.

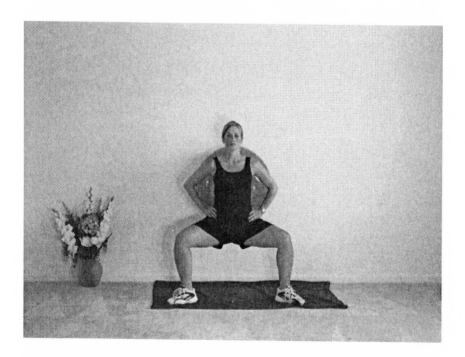

CHAPTER EIGHT

Dumbbell Training

Major muscles worked - Biceps

1. Biceps Curls - Stand with feet together, knees soft, and belly pulled in. Your arms should be straight, elbows tucked into your sides, and your palms facing forward. Inhale, then on the exhalation, squeeze the biceps and raise the dumbbells up to the shoulder. Slowly lower down to the start position. You can do one arm at a time. Do 2 or 3 sets of 8-12.

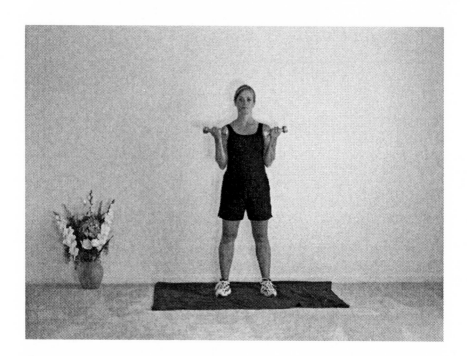

Major muscles worked - Biceps, Brachioradialis(forearm)

2. Hammer Curls - Start in the same position as the Biceps curls, only face the palms in toward your body. Repeat the same motion as the Biceps curls. Changing the hand position incorporates use of the forearm. Do 2 or 3 sets of 8-12.

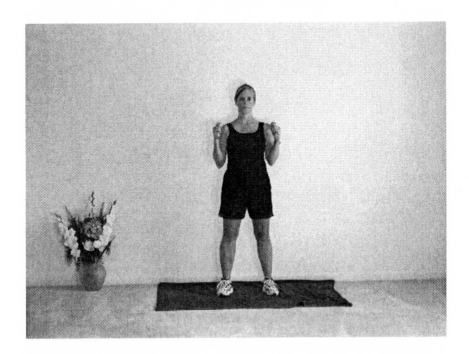

Major muscles worked - Deltoids

3. Shoulder Press - Stand with feet hip-width apart, knees soft and belly pulled in. Bring one dumbbell up to each shoulder, elbows pointing out to the side. Inhale, then on the exhalation, press the dumbbells overhead until they meet. Return to the start position. Do 2 or 3 sets of 8-12.

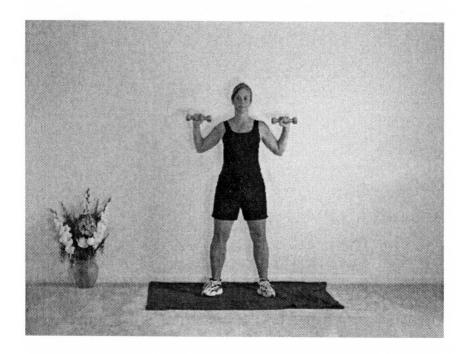

Major muscles worked - Deltoids

4. Lateral Raise - Stand with feet hip-width apart, knees soft and belly pulled in. Your arms should be hanging by your sides with a slight bend in the elbow, and your palms turned in toward your body. Inhale, then on the exhalation, raise your arms out to the sides and up to shoulder level. Lower your arms back to the start position. Do 2 or 3 sets of 8-12.

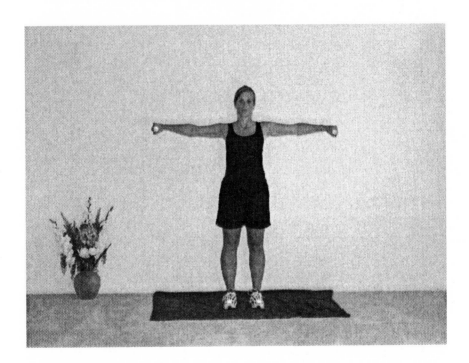

Major muscles worked - Anterior Deltoids

5. Front Raises - Stand with feet hip-width apart, knees soft and belly pulled in. Bring the dumbbells to the front of your body so that they rest against your thighs and the palms are facing down. Inhale, then on the exhalation, raise the dumbbells straight in front of you until they are at shoulder level. Lower back to the start position. Do 2 or 3 sets of 8-12.

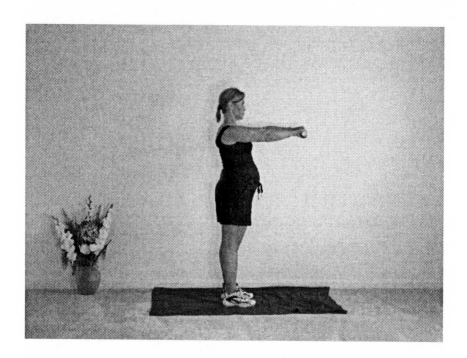

Major muscles worked - Pectorals

6. Fly - Stand with feet hip-width apart, knees soft and belly pulled in. Raise your arms up so that they form a 90 degree angle, fingers pointing up, and your upper arms are parallel to the floor. Inhale, then on the exhalation, bring the elbows and dumbbells together, squeezing the chest muscles. Open the arms back to the start position. Do 2 or 3 sets of 8-12.

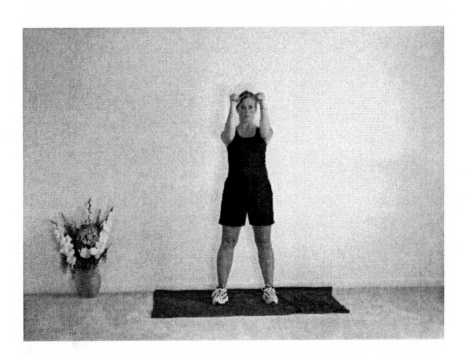

Major muscles worked - Rotator Cuff

7. Rotator Cuff Abductions - Start in the same position as the Fly, then drop the hands forward until they are parallel to the floor. Inhale, then on the exhalation, rotate the hands up so that the hands point at the ceiling. Lower down to start position. Do 2 or 3 sets of 8-12.

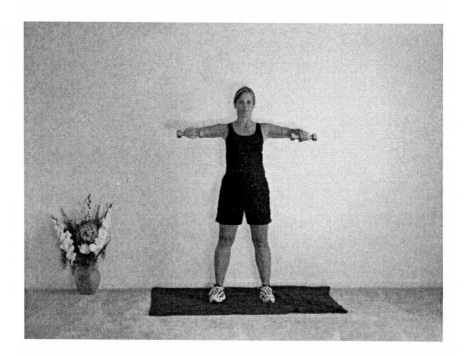

Major muscles worked - Latissimus dorsi, Triceps

8. One-arm Row/Triceps Kickback - Bring the legs to a lunge position with the left foot forward with the knee slightly bent, and the right leg straight behind you. Place your left hand on your left knee and bend at the hips slightly. The right arm should be holding a dumbbell and be extended straight down.. Keep the right elbow close to the body throughout the movement. Inhale, then on the exhalation pull the right elbow back until your upper arm is parallel to the floor. Now, extend the dumbbell backward until the arm is straight. Bend the elbow, then return to the start position. Do 1 or 2 sets of 8-12, then repeat on the left arm.

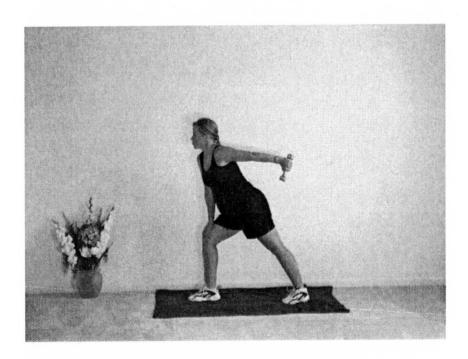

Major muscles worked - Triceps

9. Overhead Triceps Extension - Hold one dumbbell overhead with both hands, palms pointing at the ceiling. Keeping your elbows close to your ears, inhale and lower the dumbbell behind your head until the forearms are about parallel with the floor. Exhale, then return to the start position. Do 2 or 3 sets of 8-12.

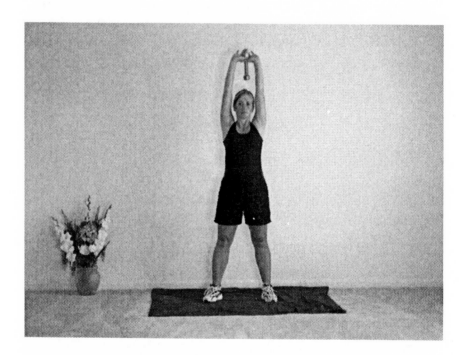

Major muscles worked - Quadriceps, Gluteals

10. Wide-leg Squats - Hold one dumbbell with both hands, arms are straight. Spread the legs wide enough apart so that when you lower down your knees will not go over your toes. Inhale as you lower your buttocks toward the floor, bending the knees until they are at about a 90 degree angle. Squeeze your buttocks, pelvic floor, and abdominal muscles. Exhale and press back up to the start position. Do 2 or 3 sets of 8-12.

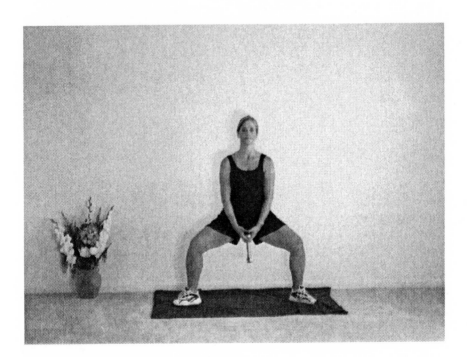

CHAPTER NINE

Body Bar

UPPER BODY

Major muscles worked - Biceps

1. Biceps Curls - Stand with feet hip-width apart, knees soft and belly pulled in. Your arms should be straight with the bar across your thighs, palms facing away from you. Keep your elbows at your sides throughout the movement. Inhale, then on the exhalation, squeeze your biceps and lift the bar up to your shoulders. Lower the bar back to the start position. Do 2 or 3 sets of 8-12.

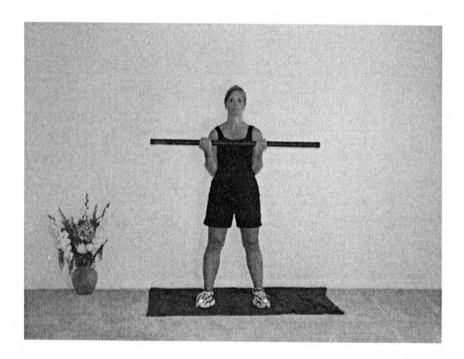

Major muscles worked - Biceps, Brachioradialis

2. Wrist Curls - Start in the same position as biceps curls. Keeping the arms straight and the bar at your thighs, inhale, then on the exhalation, curl your wrists to bring the bar slightly up toward the body. Return the bar to the start position. Do 2 or 3 sets of 8-12. This move can also be done with the palms down.

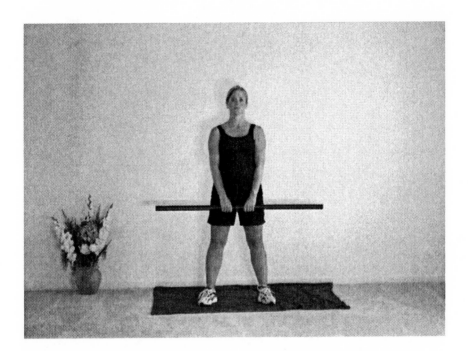

Major muscles worked - Deltoids

3. Upright Row - Stand with feet hip-width apart, knees soft, and belly pulled in. The bar should be at your thighs with the hands in an over-hand grip, a few inches apart. Inhale, and on the exhalation, bend the elbows and pull them up toward your ears until the bar reaches your chin. Lower to the start position. Do 2 or 3 sets of 8-12.

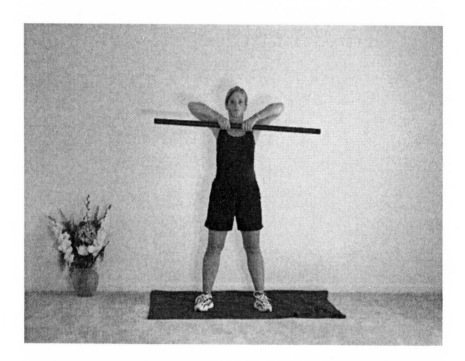

Major muscles worked - Anterior deltoids

4. Front Raise - Stand with your feet hip-width apart, knees soft, and belly pulled in. The bar should be at your thighs in an over-hand grip, hands shoulder-width apart, arms straight. Inhale, then on the exhalation, raise the bar in front of you until it reaches shoulder level. Lower to the start position. Do 2 or 3 sets of 10-12.

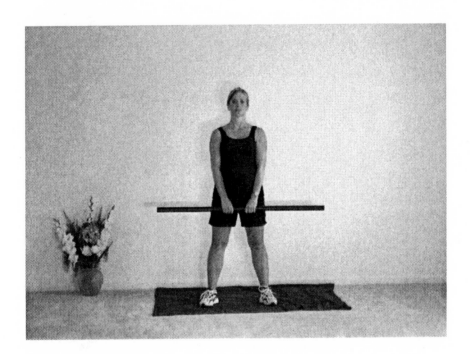

Major muscles worked - Deltoids

5. Shoulder Press - Stand with feet hip-width apart, knees soft, belly in and the bar in front of the body at shoulder level. Hands should be in an over-hand grip at the shoulders. Inhale, then on the exhalation, press the bar over your head until the arms are straight. Return the bar to the shoulders. Do 2 or 3 sets of 8-12.

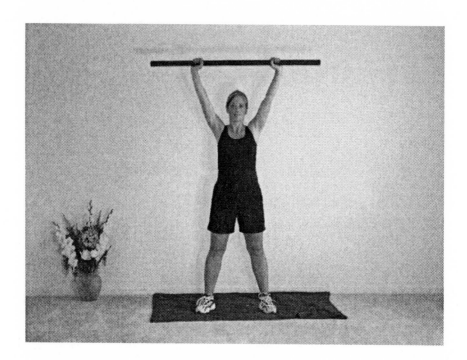

Major muscles worked - Triceps

6. Overhead Triceps Extension - Stand with feet hip-width apart, knees soft and belly pulled in. The bar should be over your head with the arms straight and shoulder-width apart with an overhand grip. Keeping the elbows stationary, inhale, as you lower the bar behind your head until your forearms are about parallel with the floor. Exhale and press the bar back up to the start position. Do 2 or 3 sets of 8-12.

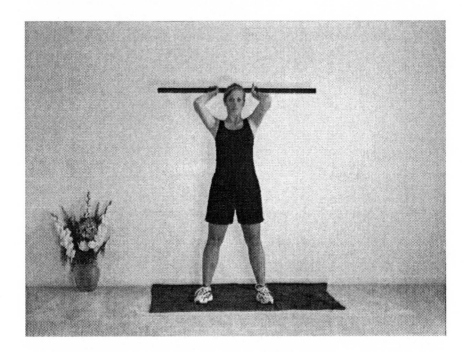

LOWER BODY

Major muscles worked - Quadriceps, Gluteals

7. Wide-leg Squats - Place one end of the bar on the floor and both hands on top of it. Open the feet wide enough apart so that when you lower down your knees will not go over your toes. Your toes should be turned out about 45 degrees. Keep your back straight and your belly pulled in throughout the movement. Inhale as you lower your buttocks toward the floor until your legs are bent about 90 degrees. Squeeze your buttocks, thighs and pelvic floor muscles, then on the exhale, press back up to the start position. Do 2 or 3 sets of 8-12.

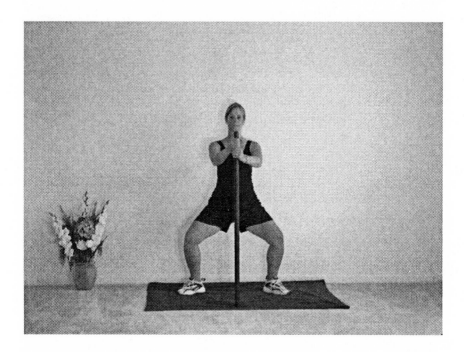

Major muscles worked - Quadriceps, Hamstrings

8. Mini Lunges - Place the bar on one end to the right side of your body with your right hand on top of it. Place your left foot 2-3 feet behind you, toes on the floor, heel raised, and leg straight. Keeping your back straight and your belly pulled in, inhale, and lower your buttocks toward the floor a few inches, bending the knees. Exhale and press through the legs back to the start position. Do 1 or 2 sets of 8-12, then repeat on the left leg.

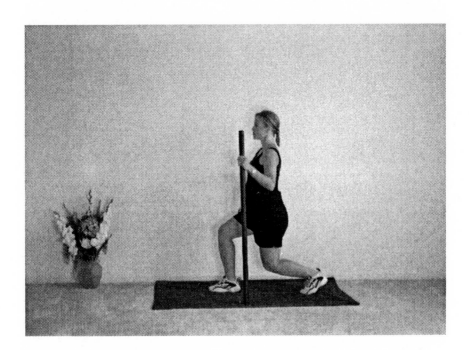

Major muscles worked - Hamstrings

9. Hamstring Curl - Place the bar on one end to the right side of your body with your right hand on top of it. Balance your weight on your right leg. Inhale, then on the exhalation, squeeze your left hamstring and pull your left heel up to your buttocks. Lower back down to the start position. Do 2 or 3 sets of 8-12, then do the right leg.

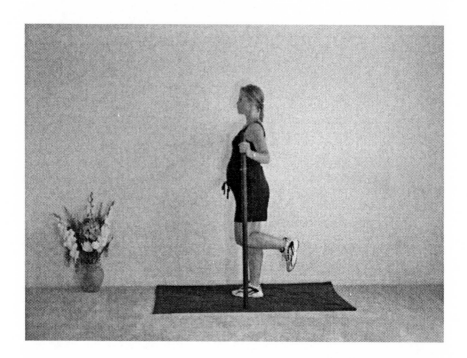

Major muscles worked - Adductors, Quadriceps

10. Front Leg Lift - Place the bar on one end to the right side of your body with your right hand on top of it. Balance your weight on your right leg. Extend your left leg straight and turn the foot out. Inhale, then on the exhalation, lift the foot off the floor until it is about even with the right knee. Do 2 or 3 sets of 8-12, then do the right leg.

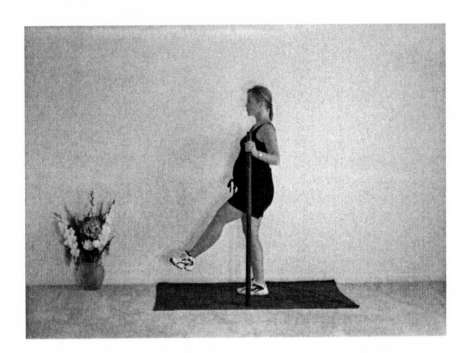

Major muscles worked - Abductors

11. Side leg Lift - Place the bar on one end to the right side of your body with both hands on top of it. Balance your weight on your right leg. Inhale, then on the exhalation, raise your straight left leg to the side and off the floor a few inches. Lower to the start position. Do 2 or 3sets of 8-12, then do the right leg.

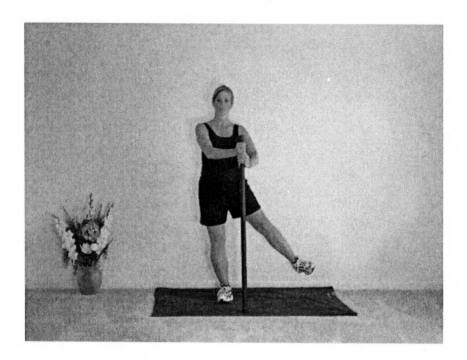

Major muscles worked - Gluteals

12. Back Leg Lift - Place the bar on one end to the right side of your body with your right hand on top of it. Balance yourself on your right leg. Inhale, then on the exhalation, raise your straight left leg behind you and off the floor a few inches. Lower to the start position. Do 2 or 3 sets of 8-12, then do the right leg.

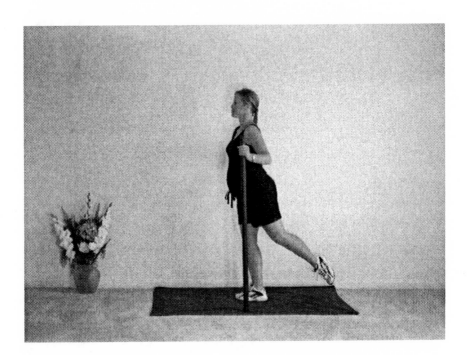

CHAPTER TEN

Exercise mat and floor exercises

EXERCISE MAT

(If you are doing #1-4 all at the same time, do all the exercises on the left leg, then do them all on the right leg to minimize turning over.)

Major muscles worked - Abductors

1. Side Leg Lifts - Lie on your right side with your head propped up on your elbow or with the right arm straight and your head resting on it. Bend the bottom leg, straighten the top leg and flex the foot. Keep the knees together. Inhale, then on the exhalation, raise the left leg 6-12 inches off the ground. Lower the leg back to the start position. Do 2 or 3 sets of 8-12, then do the right leg.

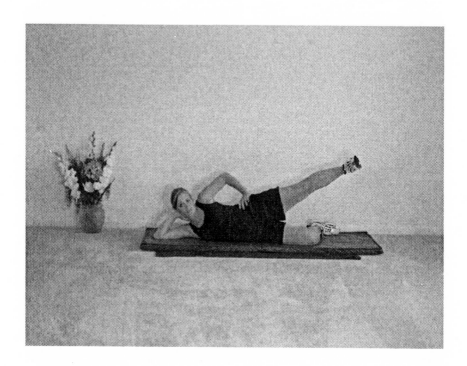

Major muscles worked - Quadriceps, Gluteals

2. Leg Press - Start in the same position as the side leg lifts. Lift the top leg up to hip level. Inhale, pull the left knee in toward your body. On the exhalation, press the left foot out until the leg is straight. Do 2 or 3 sets of 8-12, then do the right leg.

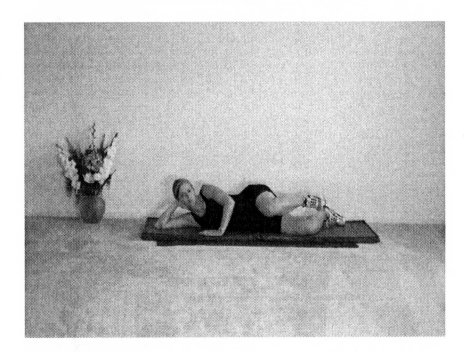

Major muscles worked - Abductors

3. Hip Abductors - Start in the same position as the side leg lifts. Bend both knees with the left on top of the right. Inhale, then on the exhalation, lift the left leg up and open the left hip until the knee points toward the ceiling. Lower the leg down to the start position. Do 2 or 3 sets of 8-12, then do the right leg. * You can keep the feet together if it is more comfortable.

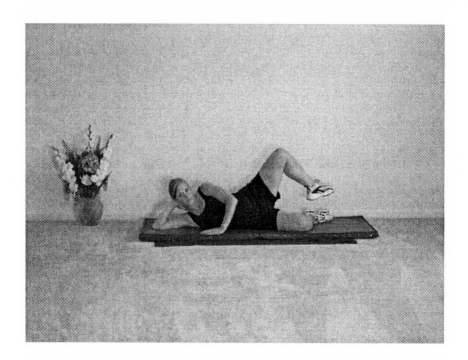

Major muscles worked - Adductors

4. Inner Thigh Lift - Start in the same position as the side leg lifts. Straighten the bottom leg and bend the top knee, bringing the foot to the floor behind you. Inhale, then on the exhalation lift the right leg off the floor a few inches. Lower the leg down to the start position. Do 2 or 3 sets of 8-12, then do the left leg. * The top foot can be placed on the floor in front of you if it is more comfortable.

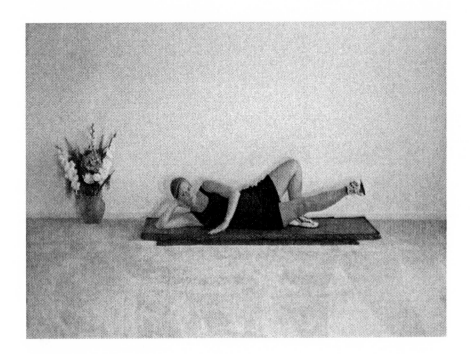

Major muscles worked - Gluteals, Hamstrings, lower and upper back,

5. Spinal Balance - Come to your hands and knees. Your hands should be directly under your shoulders and your knees should be under your hips. Inhale, and simultaneously lift and extend the right arm and the left leg until they are parallel to the ground. Exhale, and lower down to the floor. Do the other arm and leg. Do 4-8 repetitions on each side.

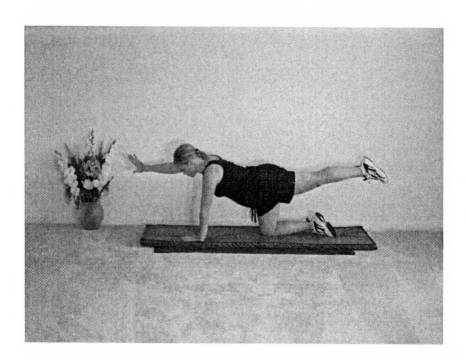

Major muscles worked - Abdominals

6. Reclining Lower Abdominal Leg Lifts - From a sitting position, place your hands or your elbows on the floor behind you, or prop yourself up on some pillows so you semi-recline. Knees should be bent with your feet flat on the floor. Contract your abdominal muscles by pulling your naval into your spine, then straighten the right leg and raise it 45 degrees. Hold for 5 counts, then lower the leg to the start position. Do 5-10 times on each leg either simultaneously or alternately.

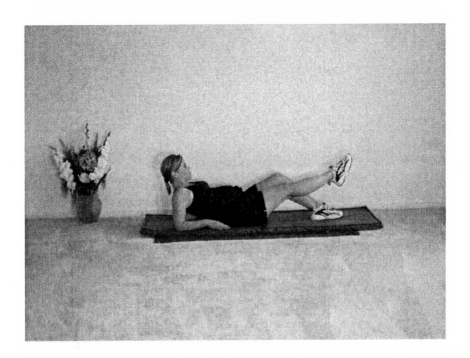

AT THE WALL EXERCISES

Major muscles worked - Pectorals, Deltoids, Triceps

1. Push-ups - Stand facing a wall with your feet 1-2 feet away from it. Place your hands on the wall slightly wider then shoulder-width apart. Keep your belly pulled in and your back straight. Inhale, bend your elbows and bring your chest toward the wall until your nose almost reaches it. Exhale and return to the start position. Do 2 or 3 sets of 8-12.
   * The farther your feet are away from the wall, the more difficult the exercise will be.

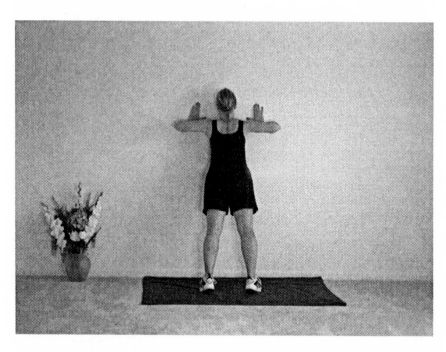

Major muscles worked - Hamstrings

2. Standing Leg Curls - Stand facing a wall with your toes a few inches away from it and your hands on the wall shoulder-width apart. Keep your belly pulled in and your back straight. Balance your weight onto your right leg. Inhale, then on the exhalation squeeze your left hamstring and pull the left heel up to your buttocks. Return the foot to the start position. Do 2 or 3 sets of 8-12, then do the right leg.

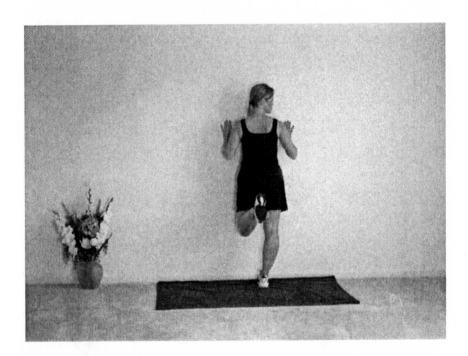

(#3-5 can be done in order on the left leg, then the right leg)

Major muscles worked - Adductors, Quadriceps

3. Front Leg Lift - Stand sideways next to a wall, arms length away, with your right side facing it. Place your right hand on the wall for support, and place your left hand on your left hip. Keep your belly pulled in and your back straight. Balance your weight on your right leg and turn your left foot out about 45 degrees. Inhale, then on the exhalation, raise your straight right leg off the floor a few inches. Lower the leg to the start position. Do 2 or 3 sets of 8-12, then do the left leg.

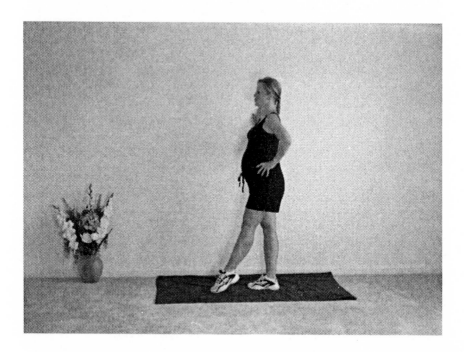

Major muscles worked - Abductors

4. Side Leg Lift - Start in the same position as #3. Balance your weight on your right leg. Inhale, then on the exhalation raise your left leg straight to the side and up off the floor a few inches. Lower the leg to the start position. Do 2 or 3 sets of 8-12, then do the right leg.

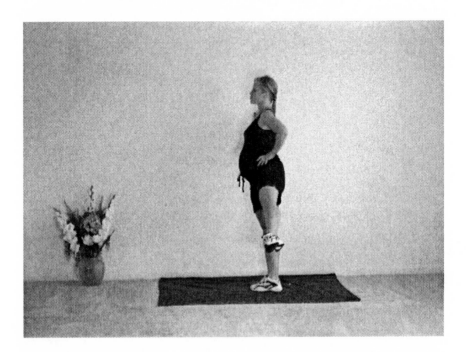

Major muscles worked - Gluteals

5. Back Hip Extension - Start in the same position as #3. Balance your weight on your right leg. Turn your left foot out to the side about 45 degrees. Inhale, then on the exhalation extend your left leg straight behind you and raise it a few inches off the floor. Lower the leg to the start position. Do 2 or 3 sets of 8-12, then do the right leg.

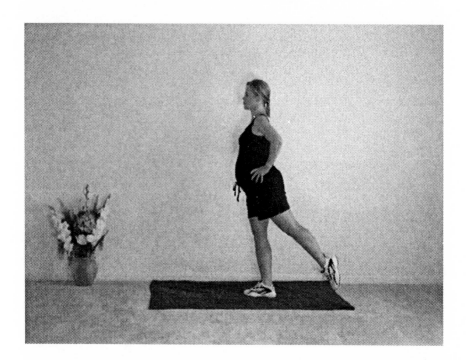

Major muscles worked - Quadriceps, Hamstrings, Gluteals

6. Plie' Squats - Stand sideways with one hand on the wall. Spread your legs wide and angle the toes out. Keep your belly pulled in and your back straight. Inhale, lower your buttocks down toward the floor until knees are bent about 90 degrees. Exhale and stand push back up to the start position. Do 2 or 3 sets of 8-12. * You do not have to lower down to 90 degrees if it is not comfortable for your knees.

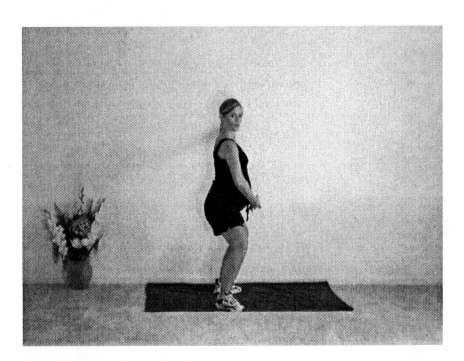

CHAPTER ELEVEN

Stretches

1. Overhead Triceps Stretch - Extend the left arm up over your head. Bend the elbow and place your left hand between your shoulder blades. Grab the left elbow with your right hand and gently pull it to the right. Hold for 10-15 seconds, then do the right arm.

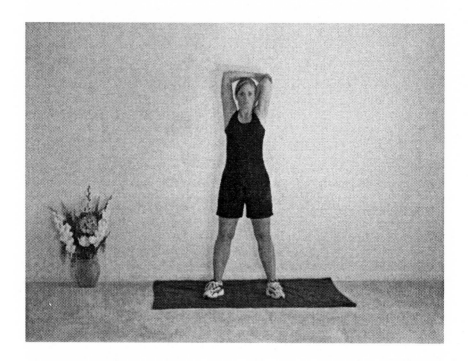

2. Shoulder and Upper Back Stretch - Bring the right arm across the chest. Grab the right arm just above the elbow with your left hand. Gently pull the right arm toward the body. Hold for 10-15 seconds, then do the left arm.

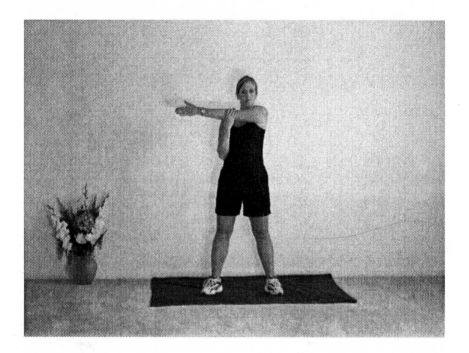

3. Chest Expansion - Clasp your hands together at your lower back. Straighten the elbows and press out the chest, squeezing the shoulder blades together. Hold for 10-15 seconds.

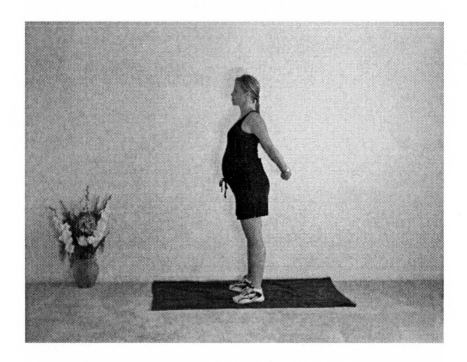

4. Seated Side Leg Stretch - Sit with your left leg extended out to the left side and your right foot pulled in by your groin. Reach down the left leg until you feel light tension under the leg. Reach the right arm up, and then lean over to the left gently. Hold for 10-15 seconds, then do the right leg.

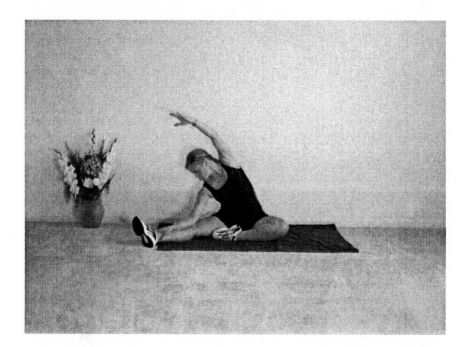

5. Straddle Stretch - Sit with your legs wide apart, hands on the floor in front of you. Hinge forward at the hips and walk your fingertips forward until you feel a gentle stretch underneath the legs. Hold for 10-15 seconds.

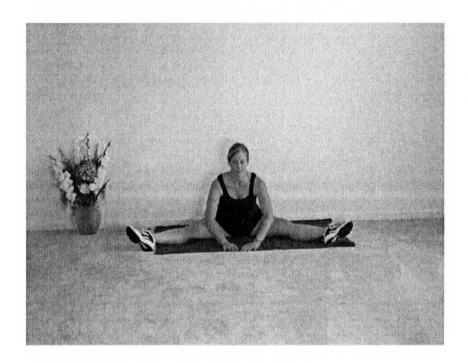

6. Cat/Cow - Come to your hands and knees. Hands should be under your shoulders, knees under your hips. Inhale, raise your head and chest up. On the exhale, drop your head down, round your back and pull your belly in. Repeat 5 or 6 times.

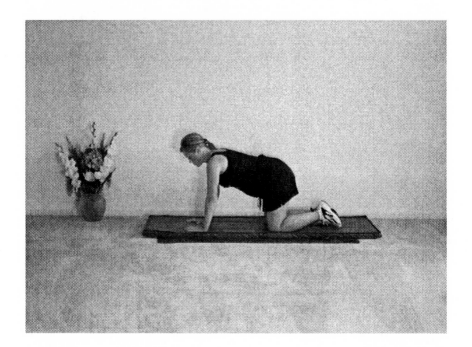

CHAPTER TWELVE

Bed-rest exercises

Occasionally situations arise that require your doctor to place you on bed-rest during your pregnancy. This does NOT mean that you have to lie perfectly still 24 hours a day and do nothing! You can spend some of this time doing beneficial exercises and stretches. In this chapter I will list for you some exercises and stretches that have already been mentioned in this book - they just may need to be modified slightly. Please ask your doctor about the exercises you choose before you begin - every situation is unique.

Exercises from:

Chapter 7 - Exercise Band

Do these exercises sitting on your bed

1. One-arm shoulder press(grab the band behind your back and adjust the resistance)
2. Triceps Extension(grab the band behind your back)
3. Lat pull-down
4. Fly

Chapter 8 - Ball

Do these exercises sitting on your bed

1. Abdominal contractions(can be done in any position)
2. Kegels(can be done in any position)
3. Leg lifts

Chapter 9 - Dumbbells

Do these exercises sitting on your bed

1. Biceps curls
2. Hammer curls
3. Shoulder press
4. Lateral raise
5. Front raise
6. Flys
7. Rotator cuff abduction
8. Overhead triceps extension

Chapter 11 - Mat

Do 1-4 on your side, #5 sitting

1. Side leg lifts
2. Leg press
3. Hip abductors
4. Inner thigh lift
5. Reclining lower ab lifts

Chapter 12 - Stretches

1. Overhead triceps stretch
2. Shoulder and upper back stretch
3. Chest expansion
4. Seated leg stretch
5. Straddle stretch
6. Cat/cow

LIST OF SOURCES

- Gallo, Birgitta, *Expecting Fitness*, (Renaissance Books, 1999)

- Somer, Elizabeth, *Nutrition for a Healthy Pregnancy*, (Henry Holt & Company, 2002)

- YMCA of the United States with Thomas W. Hanlon, *Fit for two*, (Human Kinetics, 1995)

About the Author

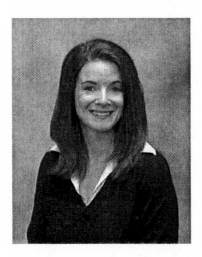

Kim Cecchi is a certified and experienced personal trainer who specializes in prenatal fitness and prenatal yoga.

During her own pregnancy with her son, Nicholas, she had some complications that restricted her physically. It made her realize how important it is to keep yourself fit during your pregnancy, and has dedicated herself to helping other women remain fit during and after their pregnancies.

She believes that even though you have limitations while you are expecting, that there are lots of options for you and she shares them with you in this book.

Kim lives in Illinois with her husband and son.

Printed in the United States
57420LVS00003B/259